CAREERS IN

SPEECH-LANGUAGE PATHOLOGY

COMMUNICATIONS SCIENCES AND DISORDERS

HEALTHCARE PROFESSIONAL

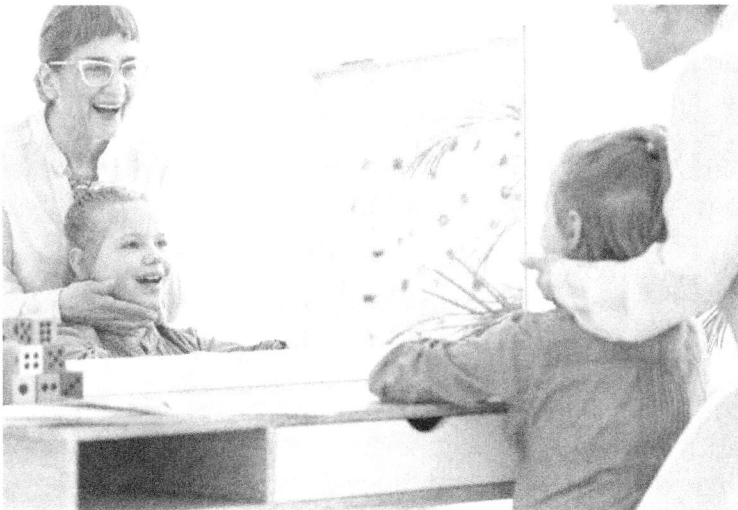

AS A CAREER FIELD, "COMMUNICATION" is generally assumed to include career paths as diverse as journalism, public relations, creative writing and even theatre. What about communication at the most essential level of speech?

Speech-language pathologists, often known as SLPs, are the dedicated professionals who help people who have trouble speaking clearly to find their voice and communicate effectively with the world around them. They are the most numerous careerists in the field of communications sciences and disorders, which also includes audiologists and scientists who study speech and hearing problems. Many people suffer from speech problems. About half of the 180,000 speech-language pathologists in the US are employed by schools to help children born with speech impairments to overcome them. The other half of speech-language pathologists work in clinics and hospitals to help people who have suffered trauma or disease, to regain their ability to communicate via speech. People who suffer strokes, for example, often lose much of their ability to speak and need intensive therapy to regain it. Speech-language pathologists also help people with swallowing disorders, which are often the result of injury or illness.

Although most speech-language pathologists choose to work for large institutions like schools and hospitals, some take an entrepreneurial leap and open their own specialty clinics, hiring other speech-language pathologists and support staff. Typically, they do not take this step until they have spent a few years working somewhere else, learning the profession, and building a reputation.

WHAT TO DO NOW

GETTING ACTUAL EXPERIENCE IN SPEECH-LANGUAGE pathology while you are still in school is not easy, but there are a few things you can do to get started in your career. Regulations vary by state, but you may be able to volunteer as an assistant to the SLP at your school or at a clinic. Some states require speech-language pathologist assistants to possess at least an associate degree in the subject in order to become official speech-language pathologist assistants, while others do not regulate support personnel at all. At this stage, however, you are not looking for an actual job, so offer your services as an unofficial – and unpaid – helper for a working speech-language pathologist. Just being around an actual professional in the field will be very informative.

An easier route may be to talk to a friend or fellow student who is working with an SLP to overcome speech and hearing impediments. Ask what it is like to have an impediment and what the SLP does to help overcome it. Most people are very sensitive about speech and hearing impediments and are painfully aware of the problems they cause in public. If you decide to approach another person with a speech or hearing impediment, first be sure that they are seeking therapy from a speech-language pathologist, and then explain that you are considering pursuing a career in the field. Show a genuine interest in their circumstance and what they are doing to make it better. Approaching a friend will almost certainly be easier than approaching a stranger.

A fun way to learn something about how speech is created by the muscles of the mouth and throat is by learning to mimic accents. Can you do a posh British accent? How about a Cockney or Irish accent? You can also try speaking English with a wide variety of foreign accents. Pick a few and see if you can mimic them. There are videos on the internet that will show you how. When you get the sound right try to slow it down and figure out exactly what you are doing with your tongue, your nose and your throat. This is what speech-language pathologists do. In fact, there are speech-language pathologists in Hollywood who teach actors how to do accents and maximize their vocal talents.

HISTORY OF THE CAREER

ALTHOUGH IT TOOK MANY CENTURIES to gain its current name and professional status, what we now call speech-language pathology has been practiced in one form or another since the dawn of civilization. Go back far enough, before the advent of written language, and speech was the only means of communication.

This is not to say that ancient cultures made great efforts to help people with speech impediments. Quite the contrary, in fact. Many ancient cultures shunned people with disabilities. Some even put to death people with serious handicaps or infirmities, either because they thought their quirks were evil or because they wanted to keep their people pure and strong. Western cultures have mostly moved beyond punishing people for problems beyond their control. Nowadays we try to help.

Thousands of years ago, nobody knew how to treat speech impediments. Lisps, stutters and other problems were regarded as unfortunate, and their sufferers were generally relegated to the fringes of society. People with a flair for speech, however, were actively cultivated and pushed to the forefront. Singers, orators, actors and storytellers were highly prized in societies without a written language or in which few people could read. Ancient Rome had a written language – Latin – but a high degree of illiteracy and no printing presses, which would not be introduced until the 1500s. The only way to get the news to the people was through town criers – people with powerful, highly trained voices who declaimed the news of the day in town squares and other busy places. Town criers were chosen for their natural speaking talents.

It took a long time before any serious efforts were put into fixing speech impediments. Among the earliest physicians to tackle speech problems was Saint Blaise, a bishop who lived in Armenia in the fifth century. Saint Blaise specialized in diseases of the throat, apparently with some success. Unfortunately, Saint Blaise was executed by a Roman governor sent to Armenia to kill all Christians. He is still remembered today by the Blessing of the Throats, a ritual carried out in many countries in conjunction with his feast day every February third.

Several European pioneers began to tackle speech impediments starting in the 1200s. Italian physician Taddeo Alderotti hypothesized that speech problems were caused by "humors," or imbalances in the moisture and vapors that connected the brain to the tongue. A few years later, fellow Italian Peter of Abano was among the first to describe how the mouth and tongue work together to articulate speech.

By the 18th century, speech therapy had evolved quite a bit. Some physicians experimented with therapy that involved delivering electrical shocks to the tongue. This method delivered some positive results, but only for a few minutes and was quite dangerous if not administered properly. Others concentrated on strict lessons in elocution in order to replace speech impediments with better muscle movement. This method is still widely used today, although it has been greatly refined.

Speech therapy started to become a recognized profession in the late 19th century. Several factors contributed to this process. Urbanization and advances in agricultural technology meant that fewer people were required to be available for farming jobs, enabling more people to pursue formal education. Society also softened its appraisal of people with disabilities – at least a little – often choosing to find solutions to their problems rather than lock them away and pretend they did not exist. The greater demand for education led to what is often called the "elocution movement," in which therapists coached people in public speaking, then considered a necessary skill for the well-educated. A few, including Alexander Graham Bell, inventor of the telephone, branched out into helping people with speech impediments.

By the 20th century, speech therapy was a recognized field. One of its most famous patients was King George VI of the United Kingdom. A naval officer by training, Prince Albert became King George VI in 1936 when his older brother Edward abdicated the throne to marry an American divorcee, which was then against the rules for British sovereigns. The new king suffered from a stutter, however. A speech impediment was not considered appropriate for a king and severely limited George VI's ability to make speeches and address his subjects on the radio, which were especially important during World War II from 1939 to 1945. Working with an Australian speech therapist named Lionel Logue, the king largely – but never completely – overcame his stutter and rallied his people to the wartime cause. He is remembered today as a hero of the war, something that would not have been possible without the help of a dedicated speech therapist. His story was immortalized in the 2010 movie *The King's Speech*, which won that year's Oscar for Best Picture.

Speech-language pathology in the United States took a great leap forward in 1925. Members of the National Association of Teachers of Speech were gathered in New York City to discuss their trade, which consisted primarily of coaching for debate and theater. Some members, however, wanted to build upon a growing trend in their field, and establish an association devoted to "scientific, organized work in the field of speech correction." By the time their meeting was over they had founded the American Academy of Speech Correction, now known as the American Speech-Language-Hearing Association, or ASHA. The ASHA claims nearly 200,000 members and is the primary source of professional certification and training for speech-language pathologists and audiologists in the United States.

Speech-language pathology is now a recognized component of most public education systems in the United States and an equally important part of the therapeutic process for adults recovering from trauma or suffering from cognitive disabilities. Career opportunities are exceptionally promising, with the field expected to grow rapidly in the coming years. This is good for you, and it is also good for society. Speech impediments are no longer treated as unfortunate and embarrassing. They are problems to be solved by dedicated professionals. You can be one of them.

WHERE YOU WILL WORK

THERE ARE NO GEOGRAPHIC LIMITATIONS on where you can work as a speech-language pathologist. Demand for these services is widespread in the United States and around the world. About half of speech-language pathologists are employed by schools. The other half work in hospitals, clinics, nursing homes and universities. About five percent of speech-language pathologists are self-employed and run their own clinics or consultancies.

Most schools in the United States have an SLP on staff, and maybe an audiologist. Some have a roving SLP who works for the school district and goes to a different school each day. Speech-language pathologists are especially important from kindergarten through high school because speech impediments are most easily treated in youth. If new habits can be inculcated when the patient is still very young, the odds are very good that they will stick for the long haul. Speech-language pathologists working in schools often work in conjunction with classroom teachers and other specialists to devise personalized educational programs for students with special needs. They usually work with students on a one-on-one basis but may also do presentations to classrooms to explain what they do and determine if there are other students who need their help. Most SLPs who work in public schools have master's degrees in the subject, although many school districts will hire SLPs with bachelor's degrees as long as they plan to pursue a higher degree in the near future.

Speech-language pathologists who work in hospitals and clinics tend to specialize in treating adults and people who have suffered trauma that has affected their speech or ability to swallow. Many dementia patients, for example, require speech therapy in order to maintain their speech as dementia progresses. So do victims of trauma, like auto accidents, who have suffered injury to their face or neck. Being a speech-language pathologist in this setting can be quite a challenge, with patients requiring a completely different approach to their unique problem. Many speech-language pathologists who work in this environment earn PhD degrees in the subject.

Speech and hearing scientists who work in universities tend to concentrate on research to learn more about the subject. They may spend time in clinical settings gathering data or assessing new techniques. They may also go far afield and work with colleagues from around the world on humanitarian missions in places where speech-language pathologists are few and far between. Essentially all speech-language pathologists who go into research at the university level have PhD degrees in speech and hearing science or earn them shortly after taking their positions.

DESCRIPTIONS OF WORK DUTIES

Education, Healthcare, Research

Speech-language pathologists do many different things. They work hard to correct a wide variety of problems with speech, communication and swallowing. To get a better idea of what speech-language pathologists do it helps to understand the scope of the issues they deal with.

According to ASHA, speech language pathologists "work

to prevent, assess, diagnose, and treat speech, language, social communication, cognitive-communication, and swallowing disorders in children and adults." That is an expansive definition. For example, speech-language pathologists are the professionals responsible for correcting difficulties in swallowing, known as dysphagia. While we normally take it for granted, swallowing is critically important to a healthy life. In addition to making speech difficult, swallowing problems can create challenges for eating. Swallowing problems can be genetic or, most often, the result of illness, injury or stroke. People of all ages suffer from swallowing problems, from kids in elementary school to senior citizens living in nursing homes.

Speech-language pathologists also work to treat communications disorders in which speech is only part of the problem. Social communications disorders involve problems with verbal and nonverbal communication. People on the autism spectrum typically display some degree of social communications disorder, and so do those suffering from traumatic brain injuries. Most people do not think too much about simple social communication. They know how to go through the basic steps of meeting somebody new, for example, or asking questions of a salesperson in a store. Many people with social communications disorders have a hard time with simple communication. They may know they have to say certain things, for example, but have difficulty saying them in the right order. They may speak in ways that are inappropriate for the setting or use body language that does not reflect their verbal communication.

Closely related to social communications disorders are language disorders in which people have a hard time expressing complex ideas or understanding others in both spoken and written language. Speech-language pathologists can solve many of these problems.

Cognitive communications disorders have become more common in recent years because people are living longer and stand a greater chance of suffering from dementia or strokes late in life. In young patients, cognitive communication disorders are usually associated with other intellectual disabilities. In either case, speech-language pathologists are a big part of the solution to helping people with cognitive communications disorders lead happier, healthier lives.

Some speech-language pathologists even help people who do not have any communications disorders but simply want to improve their speech. Actors, singers and public speakers often seek assistance from speech-language pathologists to polish their skills. Many speech-language pathologists in Hollywood earn their living teaching actors how to mimic accents for roles in movies and television programs.

In all of these roles, speech-language pathologists work to identify, diagnose and treat speech disorders, communication problems and swallowing disorders. This can involve working closely with professionals in other fields to create holistic treatments that work to solve many problems at once.

About half of speech-language pathologists are employed by schools and deal primarily with children. Most of the other half are employed by hospitals and specialty clinics. A few own their own clinics or private practices. The remainder are engaged in research, mostly in universities. All certified speech-language pathologists possess a master's degree, while those who go on to run clinics or conduct university-level research earn a professional doctorate Doctor of Clinical Science (CScD) degree or PhD in research. Most speech-language pathologists are employed full time, but high demand for their services allows many careerists to work part time or on call.

Supervising Speech-language Pathologist

Supervising speech-language pathologists are certified by ASHA to supervise other speech-language pathologists in complex work environments. To earn this certification SLPs must be fully certified in the state where they are working and have at least two years of professional experience after earning basic ASHA certification. There is also a continuing education requirement.

Supervising SLPs are senior leaders in work environments involving multiple speech-language pathologists, like clinics, private practices, hospital departments and school districts with large speech-language programs. A supervisory certificate is not equivalent to a doctoral degree. It has more to do with basic personnel management than with clinical expertise. Supervisory certification is an excellent choice for careerists who want to take charge of a complex organization and guide it to great things.

Speech-Language Pathology Technicians and Assistants

Speech-language pathology technicians and assistants are the entry-level careerists of the field. Most go on to earn full certification as speech-language pathologists but some are content to stay in secondary roles. This can be a great way to start your career in the field.

The American Speech-Language-Hearing Association defines technicians and assistants differently. A technician, sometimes known as an aide, works under the supervision of an ASHA-certified speech-language pathologist. There are no formal educational requirements or certifications to become a technician, although the ASHA assumes that technicians will have completed some degree of formal education and on-the-job training before they start working for certified speech-language pathologists. Most speech-language technicians have earned a bachelor's degree in the field and work as technicians while they earn the master's degree that will allow them to seek certification as a full-fledged speech-language pathologist.

Speech-language pathology assistants are typically careerists who have completed their master's degree and clinical studies but have not yet become fully certified by ASHA. Gaining full certification can be a demanding process. In addition to earning a master's degree and completing a clinical practicum, candidates for certification must achieve a passing score on the Praxis exam. Like many professional exams, the Praxis exam is very difficult. The ASHA recommends that careerists not take the exam until the year after they have completed all of the other requirements for certification and have been working as an assistant to a certified speech-language pathologist. Many careerists take the Praxis exam several times before they pass it.

Although you may be in a hurry following completion of graduate school to become a fully certified speech-language pathologist, do not feel compelled to run full-speed into the Praxis test. The odds of failure are very high and an early failure could damage your enthusiasm for the project. Take advantage of the opportunity to work alongside a certified speech-language pathologist for a year or so while you study for the exam.

Audiologist

Although not speech-language pathology, audiology is a related profession also governed by the ASHA. Audiologists often work in conjunction with speech-language pathologists. They just specialize in a different part of the anatomy.

Audiologists help people who have problems with their hearing or balance. Both functions are governed by the inner ear, which is also linked to the nose and throat. You have probably taken an audiology test. You sit in a soundproof booth, put on a set of headphones and listen to a series of pings. Every time you hear one you push a little button to let the examining audiologist know that you heard it. After a few minutes the results are tabulated and you receive a graph showing where your hearing is good and where it is not so good. This is the first step in diagnosing hearing problems.

If a patient shows signs of hearing loss, an audiologist may perform further evaluations to determine the cause and what can be done to correct the problem. Sometimes a good cleaning to remove excessive wax buildup is all that is needed. Other times recommendations from an audiologist are enough to get patients to change their ways, like turning down the music on their headphones or wearing hearing protection when using power tools.

Audiologists also recommend certain types of hearing aids to solve particular problems. The simplest hearing aids are small amplifiers inserted directly into the ear. They make ambient sounds louder so the patient can hear them. Some patients benefit from cochlear implants, little devices surgically installed near the ear that deliver small electrical impulses to the brain's hearing centers.

Audiologists also help patients to find ways to deal with hearing loss that cannot be corrected. Sign language, lip-reading and computer-based applications can help the hard- of-hearing to understand the world around them. As a bonus, audiologists can also help people with balance problems like vertigo.

Audiologists work in schools, clinics, hospitals and laboratories. Many go into the hearing aid business, which can be quite lucrative. Audiologists must earn a master's degree to become certified, and many go on to earn doctoral degrees. Audiology certification is offered by the American Speech-Language-Hearing Association.

STORIES OF WORKING PROFESSIONALS

I Am a Speech-Language Pathologist in an Elementary School District

"I didn't set out to become a speech-language pathologist. I was planning on becoming a special education teacher and discovered speech-language pathology along the way. Many of my colleagues followed the same path. We're all pretty happy about it.

I always knew I wanted to be a teacher. I discovered special education when I was completing my student teaching while pursuing my bachelor's degree in education. Special education struck me as something different, as going the extra mile for students in need. Kids in special education programs have cognitive disabilities. It should come as no surprise that speech impediments are more common in children with cognitive disabilities. I discovered this early in my career as a special education teacher. Kids with cognitive disabilities have a hard-enough time getting through the day and figuring out simple things. Just figuring out what to say can be very difficult. Speech impediments only make matters worse. Usually, they can be corrected.

So I spent several years working on a master's degree in speech-language pathology. I went to school in the evenings, studied hard for the Praxis test and eventually became a certified speech-language pathologist. Luckily for me, the school district in which I had been teaching for years had an opening for a speech-language pathologist so I slipped right in.

My career with the school district illustrates the evolution of speech-language pathology as a generally accepted part of a school curriculum. When I started out I was one of two speech-language pathologists in the entire district. We were known as 'floaters' because we traveled from school to school to take care of students rather than serving students at a single school. Demand for speech-language services increased steadily during this period, and after a few years I settled down at one school.

I am not a traditional classroom teacher. My students come to me one at a time or in very small groups as an addition to their regular classes. Most kids don't need my services but those who do need personal attention. My school is a fascinating place. Located in a very diverse neighborhood in a big city, my school is home to more than 30 languages. The students at my school speak more than 30 languages at home. Everything from French to Farsi, Hindi to Hebrew, Spanish to Serbian.

I love my job because I can see little successes every day. An improved accent, a lesser lisp, a more confident stutterer, a child with cognitive disabilities overcoming at least one problem. Some days can be frustrating, to be sure, but when the day comes to retire from this job there will be no doubt in my mind that I helped to make the world a better place."

I Am a Speech-language Pathologist Technician

"I am on my way to becoming a speech-language pathologist and I am enjoying every minute. I have earned my bachelor's degree in speech-language pathology and am working as a technician for a team of certified speech-language pathologists at a private clinic while pursuing my master's degree.

I learned about speech-language pathology as a child. I had a terrible stutter when I was young. It affected everything I did. It was hard to hold conversations. I couldn't respond quickly to comments or requests. I was absolutely horrified when my teachers called on me in class, and I thought there was nothing I could do about it.

Then a dedicated speech-language pathologist showed me that my stutter could be cured. It took years of therapy and plenty of emotional ups and downs but I conquered my speech impediments once and for all. It changed my life. My self-esteem improved immeasurably. I no longer spent my days in fear of speaking up.

So when I got to college there was only one major for me: speech-language pathology! My program covered everything, including public speaking, psychology, linguistics, anatomy and physiology of speech, language acquisition, audiology, speech disorders, clinical methods and much more. I loved every minute of it. I got to spend a semester as a student teacher, too. It felt great to be back in an elementary school helping kids just like me.

At the private clinic where I work now I deal mostly with adults who have suffered trauma or age-related issues like dementia or stroke. Working with the very elderly is a relatively new specialty. In the past most people didn't live long enough to suffer from dementia and stroke victims usually died. Today, more people live into old age than ever before, and many of them need speech therapy to continue to lead happy lives.

My plan is to finish my master's degree in the next two years, take the Praxis exam a year or so after graduation and look for a job at a school where I can help children the same way my speech therapist helped me. I am well on my way."

"I Am a Supervising Speech-language Pathologist at a Hospital

"I supervise a team of speech-language pathologists specializing in helping trauma patients recover their speech. Our work is therapeutic in nature, just like our peers working in schools, for example, but it is also medical in a way that conventional speech therapy is not. We work with people who have suffered serious injury to their mouth, jaw or throat, or suffered brain damage that affects their ability to speak. Every case is different.

I have spent my entire career in medical settings. I worked in private clinics early in my career and then moved into hospitals. I have nothing but respect for my peers who choose to work in schools. When I finished my master's degree and became certified, however, I decided that I wanted to try something new.

You may think you know what the human body can endure, but I'm here to tell you that you have no idea. Every day I see people who have suffered trauma so extreme that I am amazed they are still alive. Automobile accidents are the primary cause of trauma, but we also get patients who were injured in work accidents, natural disasters and crimes.

There is no way to predict what will happen in cases of trauma. Two patients can suffer similar trauma in similar accidents and have completely different challenges in recovery. Age plays a part in recovery, as the elderly tend to recover more slowly than the young. There are also intangibles to be discovered along the way. Two people of the same age with the same injury will heal in different ways just because they are different people. Attitude also plays a big part. Some people become so depressed after a traumatic injury that they just give up. I have to work very hard to get them to change their minds.

As a supervising speech-language pathologist, I am in charge of deploying the team to best effect. I am responsible for scheduling and logging hours. I also keep track of vacation time and training. I play a role in hiring and firing, too. My managerial duties do cut into my speech-language pathology time, but I don't mind."

"I Own a Speech-language Pathology Clinic

"I always wanted to be my own boss. Speech-language pathology has given me that opportunity. It took a long time to get here, but I wouldn't change a thing.

I started my career in an elementary school, like most speech-language pathologists do. I learned a lot, and then moved on to become a supervising speech-language pathologist at a hospital. I liked being the boss. It was empowering to be in charge of something bigger than myself.

After a few years in the hospital practice, I decided I had the skills necessary to run a private practice. I spent months going through the checklist on the ASHA's website for speech-language pathologists who are considering starting a practice of their own. With a combination of savings and loans from friends, I opened my practice two years ago.

I have never regretted my decision for an instant. I now employ a team of four full-time speech-language pathologists and have a long list of consultants I can call upon when necessary. I spend most of my time engaged in running the business side, but that's okay. I still get the same feeling of satisfaction I did when I was doing the speech therapy myself. I thought about pursuing a Master of Business Administration degree but have not followed through. I have taken a few business classes, though. Marketing does not come naturally to me, and finance is one of those things that nobody should leave to chance. If you want to open your own practice I recommend that you wait until you have at least several years of experience under your belt and know about managing speech-language pathologists. Then you can take the time to learn about how to run a business. If you open a practice too early in your career you could easily fail.

We don't really have a specialty here. We do a little bit of everything. We take referrals from local hospitals to help out with patients recovering from trauma. We have a growing list of elderly patients recovering from strokes. I use consultants for pediatric patients who need extra time beyond what they get in their schools (most of my consultants are retired speech-language pathologists who worked in schools but who work part time).

I love my career because there are no limits on what I can do. I would never go back to working for somebody else."

I Am a Speech-language Pathology Researcher at a University

"I always wanted to go into research but I took my time to get here. I spent a few years working in schools and a hospital before I went into research. I worked on my PhD for several years while working as a speech-language pathologist. I enjoyed the combination of doing research one day and working with patients the next. Those years really cemented for me the link between the researchers and the people who put that research to use in the real world. Many people choose to go straight through their schooling, from a bachelor's degree all the way to a PhD without spending any time doing speech-language pathology in the real world with real patients. I understand the urge to get past schooling as quickly as possible but I think blending education with experience is the way to go.

I now work at a major research university and get to spend my days digging into thorny problems that nobody has been able to solve. I get to work closely with other professionals like audiologists and ear, nose and throat specialists to figure out where our skills overlap and how we can do the most good for each other. This is the kind of high-level interaction I couldn't get working in a clinic or a school.

The life of a researcher isn't for everybody. I spend a lot of time doing statistical analysis, running control studies and generally handling the drudgery that comes with doing research. Some days seem very long. There are also endless hours preparing manuscripts according to rigorous rules, dealing with university politics and competing with my fellow researchers.

I don't really teach classes in my position but I do work closely with graduate students working on dissertations and research projects. I also hire many of them to assist me with research, and I couldn't do my job without them. I am glad to say that I have helped the best students go on to bigger and better things. As a researcher at a major university a letter from me is worth a lot. That feels good, too."

PERSONAL QUALIFICATIONS

TO BE SUCCESSFUL IN THIS CAREER YOU must be compassionate. This could be said of therapists in general, all of whom spend their days helping other people to solve problems they cannot solve on their own. Patients seen by speech-language pathologists, however, can run the gamut from frustrated adults trying to overcome the effects of injury or stroke to children with cognitive disabilities who do not even understand that they need help. In order to be effective, speech-language pathologists must always remember that their patients are people who are trying their best to grapple with a difficult situation. Do you think you can keep your chin up all day, every day?

SLPs must have excellent analytical skills in order to correctly diagnose problems and recommend therapies. The ear-nose-throat anatomy is very complex and is not exactly the same from one person to the next. If it were, everybody's voice would sound the same. All therapies for a lateral lisp, for example, will have something in common but they all have to be applied to individuals with slightly different conditions. SLPs cannot treat their patients as interchangeable. They have to put time and energy into analyzing the specific problem suffered by each patient and then devise an individualized therapy to achieve the desired result.

This requires considerable creativity. Just because two diagnoses are the same does not mean that two courses of treatment will be the same. People are different and require different treatment plans. SLPs often work in conjunction with other healthcare professionals to devise the best treatment plan for each individual. This is especially true in cases of trauma, in which a patient's speech problems may be a symptom of other severe problems that require specialized treatments. Very difficult cases may require several professionals to hold regular meetings to discuss progress and make plans for the next phase of treatment. Luckily, many of your cases will be relatively simple and respond effectively to standard methods straight out of standard practice. But many will not, and that is when you will have to get your creative energies flowing.

ATTRACTIVE FEATURES

SPEECH-LANGUAGE PATHOLOGY IS A POPULAR career for many reasons. Like most healthcare professions, speech-language pathology is about helping people to lead better lives. Everybody who goes into healthcare does so at least in part because of wanting to help people. This is as true for SLPs as it is for medical doctors, dentists or anybody else who spends years earning advanced degrees that probably will not make them rich. Healthcare is a fundamentally altruistic venture, driven by people whose primary motivation is to make the world a better place, one patient at a time. There is great personal and professional satisfaction in being a part of the healthcare world.

As a speech-language pathologist you will also get to help some of the people who need it most. Many of your patients will be children with speech impediments for whom every day is a challenge. A speech impediment can weigh heavily on a child's self-esteem, affecting their confidence and their willingness to speak up and fully participate in life. They may also be teased and ridiculed by their peers. As an SLP you can do more than simply fix a speech impediment, you can turn a child's life around and send them on the path to becoming a successful adult.

You can also help adults with speech and swallowing problems caused by trauma or dementia. If you were in the prime of life and suffered an accident that left you unable to speak, an SLP who helped you to regain your power of speech would be your hero.

Speech-language pathology is a really good job. Many SLPs are employed by schools, which offer excellent job security and a pleasant working environment, usually with summer vacations. Others are employed by hospitals, clinics and universities, all of which come with their own perks. About five percent are self-employed. These entrepreneurs can work as consultants, taking one job at a time and usually get paid by the hour. This is an ideal arrangement for somebody who has other responsibilities – like children – and wants to control their time. Others establish their own clinics and hire support staffs and other speech-language pathologists. You will have plenty of options in this career.

UNATTRACTIVE ASPECTS

SPENDING ALL DAY, EVERY DAY WITH PEOPLE in distress can be very difficult. Helping people to overcome terrible problems is a wonderful way to make a living, until you cannot take it anymore. It sounds harsh, and maybe even selfish, but there is nothing easy about spending all day, every day helping people with serious problems. Even on the best of days, you will only be taking baby steps.

Furthermore, many speech pathology patients have learning disabilities or suffer from dementia or other cognitive challenges. You may think you have made progress one day only to return the next day and realize that your patient forgot everything from the day before. Some patients will not understand you at all and may not want your help. Frustration will be a part of your daily routine.

Frustration with baby steps, incremental progress, and patients who do not really understand what you are trying to do can become tiresome. It is even harder to realize that no matter how hard you try, you will always have a few patients who you just cannot help. Their trauma is too serious or their learning disabilities too severe for you to have much impact. Maybe you can solve one problem, like a swallowing issue, but not the other problems that go with it. It is not that some cases are too hard, it is that some cases are not even possible. This can be very disappointing.

No matter how hard you try, you will always encounter people who do not appreciate your efforts. Trauma patients who want desperately to regain their speech may become frustrated and angry when you cannot magically fix their problems in an instant. Your most-fraught relationships will almost certainly be with the parents of children with severe cognitive disabilities who want so badly for their children to be "normal" that they take out their frustrations on you (and teachers, other children and anybody else who does not seem to make things better). Parents of children with speech impediments but no other impairments can also be difficult, expecting you to easily fix, say, a lisp in their otherwise-perfect child. No matter how much pride you take in your work you will always have days when you wonder why you bother.

EDUCATION AND TRAINING

CAREERS IN SPEECH-LANGUAGE PATHOLOGY require a great deal of education. While it is possible to become a speech-language technician with only a bachelor's degree, all 50 states require speech-language pathologists to possess master's degrees in order to earn state licensure. There are doctoral programs for speech-language pathologists who wish to do scientific research or become leaders in their field.

All communications sciences and disorders degrees offered by American colleges and universities are accredited by the American Speech-Language-Hearing Association (ASHA), the leading professional association in the field. ASHA also offers certification for speech-language pathologists and audiologists that is recognized across the United States. Careerists must possess a graduate degree from an accredited program in order be eligible to take the certification exam. Consider this certification to be mandatory.

There is no requirement for aspiring careerists to earn a bachelor's degree in speech-language pathology or in any particular communications sciences and disorders discipline. But because there is a requirement for careerists to earn a master's degree in their subject in order to become licensed, it makes sense for those with their mind set on a career in the field to major in the subject beginning at the undergraduate level. Those who choose undergraduate majors in something else will have to take prerequisites to get into the master's programs. A typical undergraduate program in communications sciences and disorders will include courses in neuroscience, human anatomy, hearing and balance disorders, linguistics and biology, among others. Graduates will have a solid grasp of communications and swallowing disorders. Careerists who earn bachelor's degrees can start their careers as aides or technicians to licensed professionals. They can choose to stay at this level or pursue higher education to become licensed themselves, perhaps while working part time as an assistant.

A master's degree is the most important academic credential for careerists in speech-language pathology or any other communications sciences and disorders field. Even if you intend to pursue a doctoral degree, the master's degree is the one that will make you an official practitioner. Most master's degrees in the field take about two years to complete and utilize a combination of academic coursework and actual clinical experience to deliver a well-rounded curriculum enabling graduates to begin working in the profession.

There are three doctoral degree options for careerists who aspire to terminal degrees. The clinical doctoral degree in speech-language pathology, or CScD, is intended for speech-language pathologists who want to become leaders in their professional community as educators, administrators or master clinicians. The research doctoral degree, or PhD, is for careerists who want to devote their careers to scientific research. For careerists interested in audiology, the Doctor of Audiology degree, or AuD, is a three- to four-year degree program designed to prepare candidates to treat hearing, balance and general auditory disorders. You do not have to decide on this path any time soon.

Specialist certificates are offered through specialty certification boards sponsored by the American Board of Child Language and Language Disorders, American Audiology Board of Intraoperative Monitoring, American

Board of Fluency and Fluency Disorders, and the American Board of Swallowing and Swallowing Disorders.

EARNINGS

CAREERISTS WORKING AS SPEECH-LANGUAGE pathologists can do well financially. These high-value professions require a great deal of education and expertise.

Most speech-language pathologists are employed by school districts, all of which maintain their own pay scales. Those pay scales can vary widely. Speech-language pathologists are likely to be paid more in New York City than in Tulsa, Oklahoma, but the cost of living in Tulsa is much less than in New York City. On average, however, speech-language pathologists straight out of graduate school with a master's degree and certification can expect to earn about $55,000 to $65,000 per year. This rate will rise over time with seniority, with some very senior speech-language pathologists earning more than $90,000 per year.

Careerists who choose to go into academics or research typically earn more than their counterparts working for school systems, with many universities paying more than $100,000 per year for qualified candidates. Academic positions also usually come with tenure, which is a guarantee of employment after you have spent a certain number of years on the job.

About five percent of speech-language pathologists go into private practice. Private practice can be an office like any doctor's office, where the pathologist meets with patients and perhaps employs support staff like administrative assistants and maybe a junior speech-language pathologist. Private practice can also take the form of consulting, in which the practitioner takes temporary jobs, usually for an hourly fee. As with all entrepreneurs, private practitioners can make more money than those employed in a school or hospital. In this profession, however, nobody goes into private practice until they have spent many years perfecting their skills by working for somebody else.

OPPORTUNITIES

YOU ARE ENTERING THIS LINE OF WORK at the right time. Demand for speech-language pathologists is expected to rise very fast in coming years. Advances in medical knowledge will drive most of the demand, resulting in a growing population of older people needing specialized care and people of all ages who need therapeutic treatment following trauma. Enhanced awareness of learning disabilities and speech impediments will also increase demand for specialized services, especially for the young.

It has often been said that two-thirds of all the people who have ever lived past the age of 65 are alive today. People are living longer than ever due to a combination of advances in medical care and in general health awareness. People today can count on lifesaving treatments that did not exist a few decades ago. They also know more about how to stay healthy than their ancestors did. This is all good news. The human body has its limits, however. More people than ever suffer from dementia, for example, a late-in-life malady that afflicted relatively few in the past because most people died of something else before dementia became a threat. Strokes are also uncomfortably common. Both conditions can result in speech, swallowing and hearing impediments that benefit from therapy.

Advances in medical knowledge also generate demand for speech pathology services for people of all ages recovering from traumatic injuries or disease. There have always been people in recovery from life-threatening events, but there are more than ever today because more people recover than ever before. People who probably would not have survived serious accidents in decades past now do survive and need specialized therapy to lead full lives. This creates opportunities for speech-language pathologists.

Advances within communications science and disorders have also boosted demand for speech and hearing therapy. Not too many years ago, many speech and hearing problems were simply dismissed as quirks some people had to learn to live with. Unfortunate, perhaps, but too difficult to solve. That is no longer necessarily the case. Parents of children with speech impediments are much more likely to seek out therapy today than just a few years ago, partly because therapies available today are more effective than those of the past, and also because the experts parents rely upon, like teachers and physicians, are more willing to recommend therapy in the first place. We now know that tackling speech impediments early in life offers the best chance of curing them. We also know that untreated speech impediments can lead to problems later in life, including lower self-esteem and the subsequent achievement deficits that come with it. Speech-language pathologists can solve more problems today than ever before.

GETTING STARTED

WHEN THE TIME COMES TO STEP OUT and look for your first professional job, step out boldly! Get your personal marketing materials in tip-top shape. A résumé may be the single-most important document you ever create. It is your calling card, your personal advertisement, your poster and your marquee all wrapped up into one. People who make hiring decisions spend an average of about 10 seconds looking at each résumé they receive. From a stack of 100 résumés, they will pick out six or eight to call for interviews. One of those lucky few will get the job. This means that your résumé has to be better than 93 percent of other resumes just to get an interview. Take the time to do it right. If you are unsure of your own résumé writing skills there is no shortage of books and apps out there to help you. There are also professional résumé writers who will help you for a fee. Your college or university may offer résumé services in its out-placement office. Take the time to prepare a traditional résumé even if most of the jobs you apply for use automated forms online. Cutting and pasting information from your résumé into boxes online is much easier than writing it from scratch every time. Also, you never know when you may need to email a traditional résumé to somebody. It pays to be prepared.

Once you have your résumé together send it to everybody you have ever met in the speech-language pathology business. Even if they do not have a job to offer you, sending them your résumé says that you are in the market and that you mean business. You never know when somebody might forward your résumé to somebody you have never met who just might have a job with your name on it. This is why it pays to make good impressions on everybody you meet. Be the candidate everybody wants to hire.

Keep an open mind. Be prepared to accept a position that is not quite your dream job if that is what it takes to get started. It is always easier to get a job when you already have a job. You will be making a reputation for yourself, networking and seeing what is out there.

You will learn a great deal in your first few years as a professional speech-language pathologist, and you may change your definition of the perfect job quite a few times before you finally find it.

ASSOCIATIONS, PERIODICALS, WEBSITES

■ **ABA Resources**
www.abaresources.com

■ **Alzheimer's Association**
www.alz.org

■ **American Academy of Private Practice in Speech Pathology and Audiology**
www.aappspa.org

■ **American Audiology Board of Intraoperative Monitoring**
www.aabiom.com

■ **American Board of Child Language and Language Disorders**
www.childlanguagespecialist.org

■ **American Board of Fluency and Fluency Disorders**
www.stutteringspecialists.org

■ **American Board of Swallowing and Swallowing Disorders**
www.swallowingdisorders.org

■ **American Speech-Language-Hearing Association**
www.asha.org

■ **Arizona Speech-Language-Hearing Association**
www.arsha.org

■ **Autism Speaks**
www.autismspeaks.org

■ **Bilinguistics**
www.bilinguistics.com

■ **California Speech-Language-Hearing Association**
www.csha.org

■ **Casana**
www.apraxia-kids.org

■ **Corporate Speech Pathology Network**
www.corspan.org

■ **Crazy Speech World**
www.crazyspeechworld.com

■ **Dysphagia Ramblings**
www.dysphagiaramblings.net

■ **Home Speech Home**
www.home-speech-home.com

■ **Illinois Speech-Language-Hearing Association**
www.ishail.org

■ **Iowa Speech-Language-Hearing Association**
www.isha.org

■ **Kidmunicate**
www.kidmunicate.com

■ **National Aphasia Association**
www.aphasia.org

■ **National Stroke Association**
www.stroke.org

■ **Pediastaff**
www.pediastaff.com

■ **San Diego State University**
www.sdsu.edu

■ **Speaking of Speech**
www.speakingofpseech.com

■ **Speech Buddies**
www.speechbuddy.com

■ **Speech-Language-Hearing Association of Virginia**
www.shav.org

■ **Speechlanguage-Resources**
www.speechlanguage-resources.com

■ **Speechpathology.com**
www.speechpathology.com

■ **Speech Science**
www.speechscience.org

■ **Speechtherapypd.com**
www.speechtherapypd.com

■ **Speech Therapy Ideas**
www.speechtherapyideas.com

■ **Start a Therapy Practice**
www.startatherapypractice.com

■ **Stuttering Foundation**
www.stutteringhelp.org

■ **Voice Medicine**
www.voicemedicine.com

■ **Wisconsin Speech-Language Pathology and Audiology Association**
www.wisha.org

CAREERS INTERNET DATABASE
www.careers-internet.org

Printed in Great Britain
by Amazon